GARLIC

MARIAN KIM

ISBN: 1508599408

ISBN-13: 978-1508599401

CONTENTS

MARIAN KIM

1

PROPERTIES

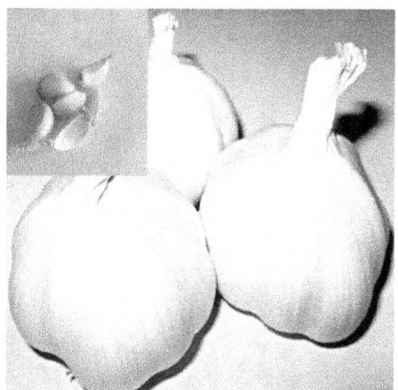

Scientific name: Allium sativum

Other names: nectar of the gods, camphor of the poor, stinking rose

Nutrients: Garlic is good source of selenium which is a potent anti-oxidant

Properties

Anti-inflammatory properties

Anti-aging properties

Anti-oxidant properties which protect the cells from the free radical damage that causes premature aging and degenerative disease.

Anti-cancer properties

Antiseptic (antibacterial, antiviral, antifungal) properties

Immune boosting properties

Garlic contains allicin which has blood pressure lowering properties, lipid lowering properties, antibacterial, antioxidant properties.

* * * * *

2

USES

Medically Proven Uses

Cancer prevention

A research review in the *American Journal of Clinical Nutrition* revealed that eating garlic lowered the rates of cancer of the ovary and colon. Garlic was also shown to reduce the numbers and size of colon polyps which are the precancerous growths associated with colorectal carcinoma. Garlic is also thought to be beneficial in preventing stomach cancers. It is also used to prevent cancers of the rectum, breast, prostate and lung. Garlic is also used to treat bladder and prostate cancer.

High blood pressure treatment

Garlic contains allicin which has blood pressure lowering properties. In a study done at the *Clinical Research Center of New Orleans* patients who had severe hypertension were noted to have reduced blood pressure on taking a garlic preparation with 1.3 % allicin. Garlic has also been used to lower high blood pressure in pregnancy, a condition which is known is pre-eclampsia.

Atherosclerosis prevention

Some studies suggest that garlic can slow the development of atherosclerosis (hardening of the arteries). However, other studies do not support these findings.

Common cold management

Garlic has antiviral properties and it is used for the common cold. A study found that people who took garlic during the cold season had fewer colds and the symptoms in those who developed them resolved faster. Garlic is also used for coughs and the flu as well as for asthma, bronchitis and infections like sinus infections.

Fungal infection treatment

Garlic has antifungal properties and is used to manage yeast infections. Garlic oil is used to treat fungal infections like ringworm, tinea cruris (jock itch) and athlete's foot. Garlic gel with 0.6% ajoene is also used to treat ringworms and jock itch. Garlic gel with 1.0% ajoene is used to treat athlete's foot and it is as effective as the prescription antifungal terbinafine.

Tick bite prevention

Garlic is used to prevent tick bites. Research has shown that people who eat large amounts of garlic over five months seem to have fewer tick bites.

Other Uses

Lowering high cholesterol

Garlic is thought to lower cholesterol since it contains allicin which has lipid lowering properties when eaten daily. Evidence from studies is conflicting.

Preventing blood clots

Garlic thins the blood and prevents clotting.

Heart disease prevention

Garlic prevents plaque formation in the blood vessels and lowers the risk of atherosclerosis by reducing the levels of homocysteine. It also prevents heart disease by lowering blood pressure and cholesterol levels, thinning the blood and acting as an anti-oxidant. Garlic is also used for coronary heart disease and heart attacks. A previous study demonstrated that fresh garlic was more potent in protecting the heart than processed garlic.

Acne treatment

Garlic has antiseptic (antibacterial) properties which are useful for managing acne. Its anti-inflammatory properties are useful for dealing with the inflammation associated with acne. Garlic also has immune boosting properties.

Diarrhea management

Garlic aids the management of diarrhea and especially traveler's diarrhea since it has antibacterial properties. It is also used for abdominal pain or stomache.

Lower blood sugar

Garlic is also thought to lower blood sugar levels in patients with diabetes though more research is required.

Benign prostatic hyperplasia (BPH) treatment

Garlic has been used for treating BPH which is an enlarged prostate gland. A study found that men with BPH who used garlic had fewer urinary symptoms and the size of the gland also reduced.

Osteoarthritis treatment

Garlic has been used to treat osteoarthritis. It is also used for gout and other causes of rheumatism.

Fever treatment

Garlic is also used to treat fever.

Hay fever treatment

Garlic has been used to treat hay fever (allergic rhinits).

Headache treatment

Garlic has been used to treat hay fever (allergic rhinits).

Hemorrhoid treatment

Garlic is also used to treat hemorrhoids.

Immune system boosting

Garlic is used to boost or build the immune system.

Stress management

Garlic is used for stress management as well as for dealing with fatigue.

Wart treatment

Garlic oil is used to treat warts and corns.

3

SAFETY PRECAUTIONS

1. Persons schedule to have surgery should not use garlic 2 weeks before and 2 weeks after the operation since it is a blood thinner.

2. Person with severe peptic ulcers should not use it as it can increase acid production.

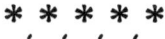

4

DRUG INTERACTIONS

1. Persons using blood thinners like coumadin (Warfarin), heparin, aspirin and other antiplatelet medications like clopidogrel (Plavix), dalteparin (Fragmin), enoxaparin (Lovenox) should avoid/not use garlic since it can also prevent clotting.

2. Persons using high blood pressure medications should avoid using/not use garlic since it can also lower the blood pressure.

3. Persons using diabetes medications should avoid using/not use garlic since it is thought to lower the blood sugar levels.

4. Persons taking isoniazid (INH) which is used to treat TB should avoid using/not use garlic since it can reduce how much isoniazid absorbed by the body and how well it works.

5. Persons taking non-nucleoside reverse transcriptase inhibitors (NNRTIs) like nevirapine (Viramune), delavirdine (Rescriptor) and efavirenz (Sustiva) which are used to treat HIV should not use garlic since it can increase how fast the body breaks them down and thus decrease their effectiveness in the body.

6. Persons taking saquinavir (Fortovase) which is used to treat HIV should not take garlic since it can increase how fast the body breaks it down and thus decrease its effectiveness.

7. Persons taking oral contraceptive pills (birth control pills) with estrogen should not take/avoid garlic since it can increase the rate at which the body breaks down the estrogen and thus decrease the effectiveness of the pills.

8. Persons taking cyclosporine (Neoral, Sandimmune) should not take garlic since it can increase how fast the body breaks it down and thus decrease its effectiveness.

9. Persons taking medications which are broken down by the liver should not take/avoid garlic since it can decrease how quickly the body breaks them down and thus increase their effects and side effects. Examples of such medications include acetaminophen, chlorzoxazone (Parafon) and theophylline.

Garlic can also increase how quickly the body breaks down some medications and thus decrease their effects. Examples of such medications include fexofenadine (Allegra), itraconazole (Sporanox), ketoconazole (Nizoral), lovastatine (Mevacor).

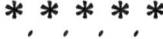

5

COOKING TIPS

Flavor: Hot onion-like

Goes well with: Meat dishes e.g. beef and pork, poultry e.g. chicken, pasta sauces, soups, stews, salad dressings, marinades

Can be substituted with: Onion

Equivalents: 1 garlic clove is equivalent to 1/8 teaspoon garlic powder

Tips: Whole garlic heads can be roasted and then removed from the skin and added to salads or spread on bread.

* * * * *

6

HERBAL RECIPES

Garlic Tablets

Equipment

Knife

***

Ingredients

Garlic cloves

***

Instructions

1. Peel the skin from the garlic cloves and cut them into two or three small pieces.

2. Swallow them with water like tablets.

***

Tips

1. Garlic tablets can also be placed between the toes and socks worn overnight in order to utilize the healing effects of garlic.

*****

Garlic Juice

Equipment

Food processor

Sieve

***

Ingredients

Garlic cloves

***

Instructions

1. Peel the skin from the garlic cloves and place them in the food processor.

2. Blend them until they become a puree.

3. Strain the puree with a sieve and collect the juice in a clean container.

***

Tips

1. Blend the garlic with fresh parsley to reduce its odor.

*****

Garlic Syrup

Equipment
Jar with airtight lid

***

Ingredients
1 cup fresh garlic juice (see above recipe)

1 cup honey

***

Instructions
1. Mix the garlic juice with the honey.

2. Store the syrup in an airtight container in the fridge.

***

Tips
1. Add a few peeled garlic cloves to make your garlic syrup more potent.

2. Garlic syrup can be used to ward off coughs and colds.

*****

Garlic Butter

Equipment

Large glass bowl

Electric mixer or stick blender or wire whisk

Molds such as ice cube trays (optional)

***

Ingredients

½ cup butter

2 tablespoons of finely minced, fresh garlic

***

Instructions

1. Place the butter in a warm place so that it can soften.

2. Put butter and garlic in a large glass bowl and blend well until thoroughly mixed.

3. Refrigerate until it hardens. You can refrigerate it in molds or ice cube trays to give it a special shape.

*****

Garlic Infused Oil

Equipment

Double boiler

Large glass bowl

Sieve and cheesecloth

Sterilized dark jars

***

Ingredients

16 fl oz. (500 ml) vegetable oil like organic olive, sweet almond oil or sunflower oil

8 oz. (250 grams) slightly bruised fresh garlic

***

Instructions

1. Place the HERB and oil in the glass bowl ensuring that the oil covers the garlic. Simmer them in a double boiler for 1 hour at around 120 degrees Fahrenheit (49 degrees Celsius). Do not let the mixture boil. You can repeat this step several times after letting the oils cool to create more concentrated herb infused oils.

2. Strain the mixture through the sieve and cheesecloth into a clean, dark jar ensuring you squeeze out as much oil as you can from the cheesecloth.

3. Label your jars and store your garlic infused oils in a cool dark place or in the refrigerator and use them within 3 months.

*****

Garlic Vinegar

Equipment

Large glass bottle with a well-fitting, non-metal lid or cork

***

Ingredients

1 quart (1 liter) white vinegar

2 tablespoons of slightly bruised fresh garlic

***

Instructions

1. Place the garlic in the glass bottle.

2. Add the vinegar and fill the bottle to ½ inch from the top ensuring all the garlic is covered by vinegar.

3. Seal the bottle and let it stand for up to 6 months. The longer it stands, the stronger the flavor becomes.

*****

Garlic Tea

Equipment

Tea pot or kettle

***

Ingredients

1 peeled garlic clove

1 tablespoon honey

1 cup of boiling water

***

Instructions

1. Put the garlic in a tea pot or kettle, add the boiling water and let it steep while covered for 10 -15 minutes.

2. Strain the tea to remove the garlic cloves and add the honey before drinking.

*****

Garlic Tincture

Equipment

Glass jar with tight fitting lid

Dark tincture bottles

Cheesecloth

***

Ingredients

14 oz (400 gm) of fresh garlic

30 oz (1 liter) of 80-100 proof vodka

***

Instructions

1. Fill 1/3 of the glass jar with the chopped garlic.

2. Add the vodka to completely fill the jar to the top.

3. Seal the jar and label it with the date of preparation and name of garlic used.

4. Store the glass jar in a dark place for 6 weeks ensuring that you shake them weekly.

5. After 6 weeks strain out the garlic with a cheesecloth and pour the tincture into dark tincture bottles.

6. Label the tincture bottles with the date and name of garlic used.

7. Store your herbal tinctures away from light and heat.

*****

Garlic Poultice

Equipment

Cheesecloth or old cotton sheet strips

***

Ingredients

1 tablespoon crushed garlic

Boiling water

***

Instructions

1. Add enough boiling water to the crushed garlic to wet it and make a thick paste.

2. Spoon the garlic paste onto the cheesecloth (or bed sheet strips) to make the poultice.

3. To use, apply the poultice to the affected area and cover with another piece of hot, wet cloth. Replace the hot, wet cloth when it cools with another hot one to keep the poultice hot.

***

Tips

1. Garlic poultice can be placed on the chest to relieve the congestion of coughs and colds.

###

ABOUT THE AUTHOR

Marian Kim is an experienced alternative medicine practitioner.

*****

OTHER BOOKS BY THE AUTHOR

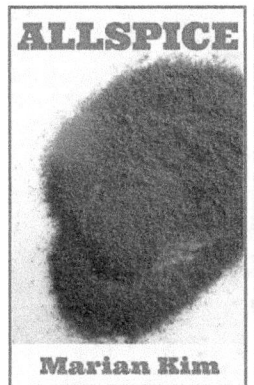

ALLSPICE

Marian Kim

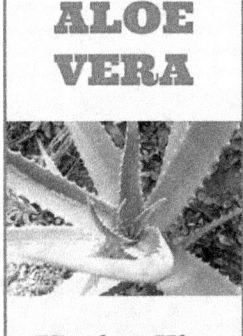

ALOE VERA

Marian Kim

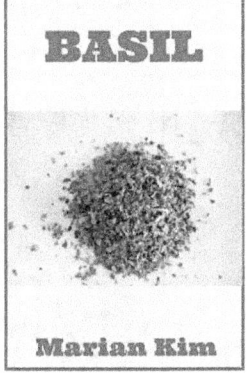

BASIL

Marian Kim

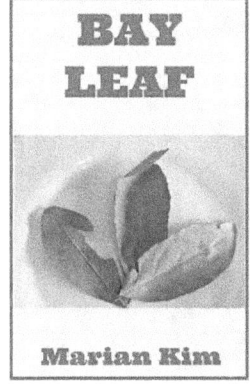

BAY LEAF

Marian Kim

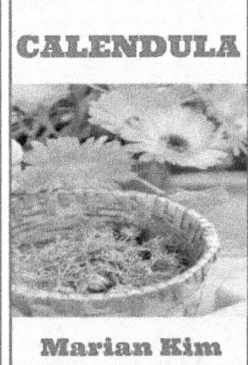

CALENDULA

Marian Kim

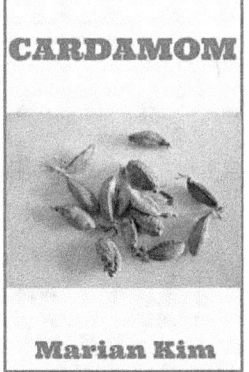

CARDAMOM

Marian Kim

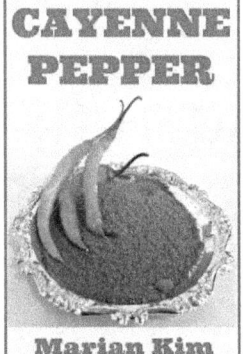

CAYENNE PEPPER

Marian Kim

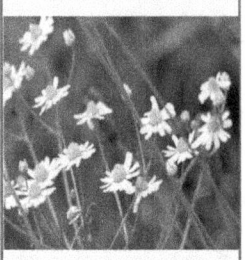

CHAMOMILE

Marian Kim

CILANTRO & CORIANDER

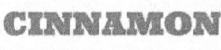

Marian Kim

CINNAMON

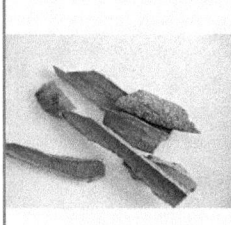

Marian Kim

CLOVES

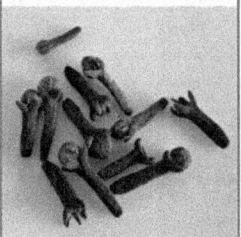

Marian Kim

CUMIN

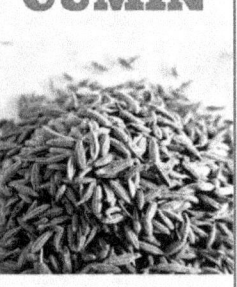

Marian Kim

DANDELION

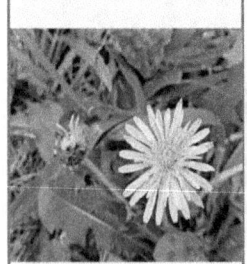

Marian Kim

DILL

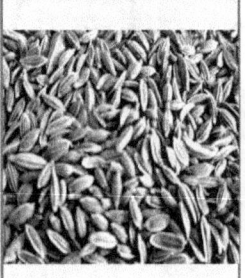

Marian Kim

ECHINACEA

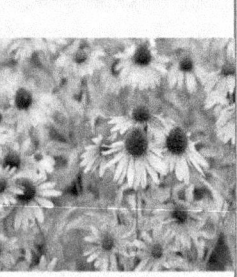

Marian Kim

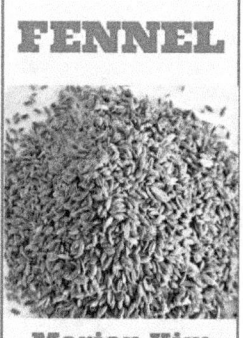

FENNEL

Marian Kim

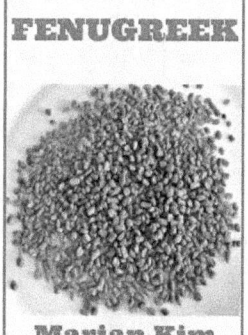

FENUGREEK

Marian Kim

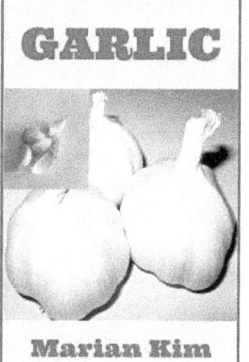

GARLIC

Marian Kim

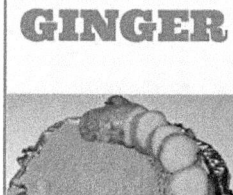

GINGER

Marian Kim

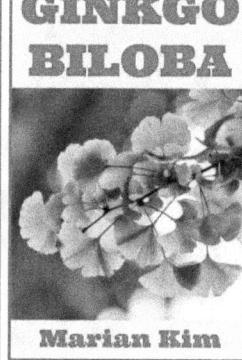

GINKGO BILOBA

Marian Kim

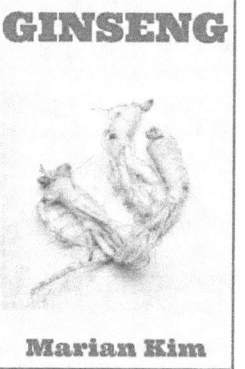

GINSENG

Marian Kim

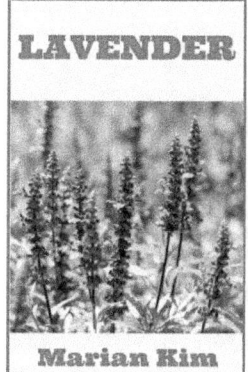

LAVENDER

Marian Kim

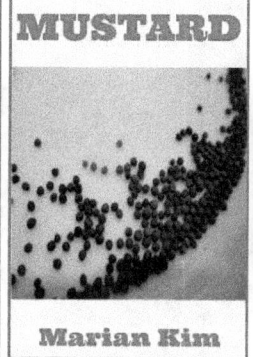

MUSTARD

Marian Kim

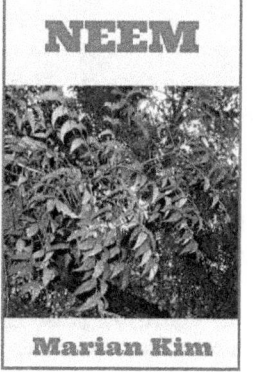

NEEM

Marian Kim

NUTMEG & MACE

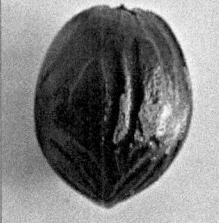

Marian Kim

OREGANO

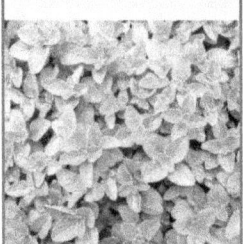

Marian Kim

PAPRIKA

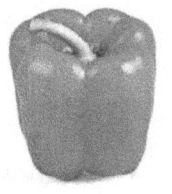

Marian Kim

PARSLEY

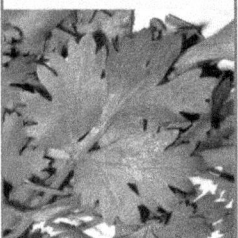

Marian Kim

BLACK & WHITE PEPPER

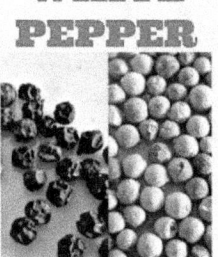

Marian Kim

PEPPERMINT

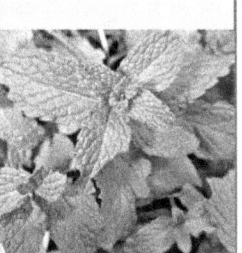

Marian Kim

ROSE HIPS

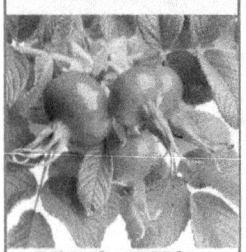

Marian Kim

ROSE PETALS

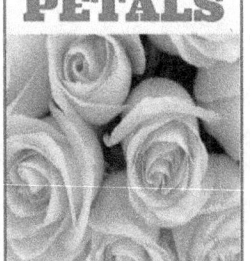

Marian Kim

ROSEMARY

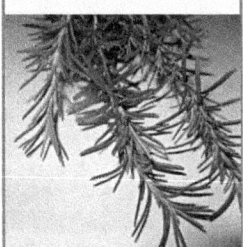

Marian Kim

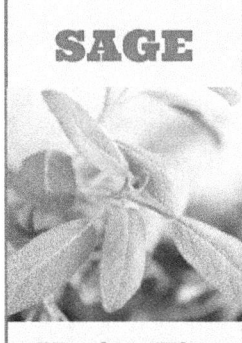

SAGE

Marian Kim

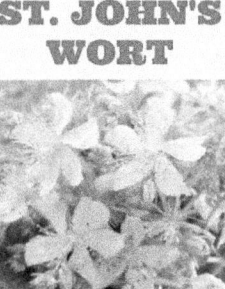

ST. JOHN'S WORT

Marian Kim

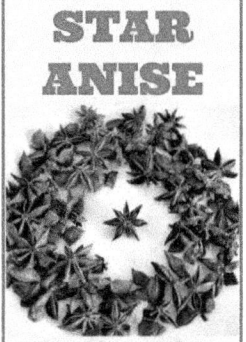

STAR ANISE

Marian Kim

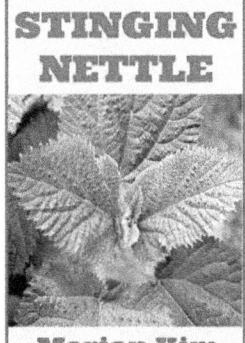

STINGING NETTLE

Marian Kim

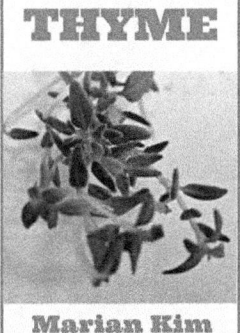

THYME

Marian Kim

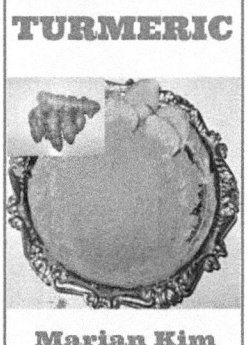

TURMERIC

Marian Kim

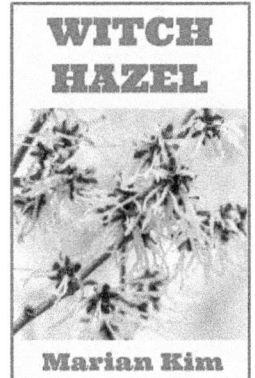

WITCH HAZEL

Marian Kim

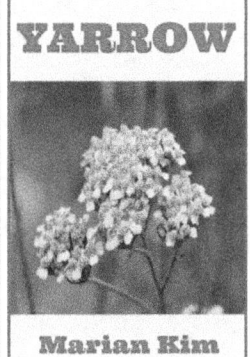

YARROW

Marian Kim

*****